Paleo:

A Beginner's Guide
Contemporary Caveman's Footpath to Radiant Health

Contents

An Introduction to the Paleo Way

Lots of people are talking about the Paleo Diet these days--how great it is for weight loss, increased energy, and better overall health (not to mention looking better naked!). However, there is, as usual, a lot of misinformation being spread around, resulting in confusion as to what the Paleo Diet really is.

The basic premise of the Paleo Diet is that the human body is ill-adapted to digest grains, legumes, and other foods which weren't eaten prior to the Agricultural Revolution. Our pre-agricultural ancestors got their food by hunting and gathering. They ate lots of meat, when it was available. They ate fruits, berries, nuts and seeds, and whatever non-poisonous plants they could find in their particular environments.

Archeological and anthropological data suggest that humankind was largely free from the ills that plague our modern Westernized societies, including obesity, cancer, cardiovascular and autoimmune diseases. Modern molecular biology, immunology and endocrinology support this observational data.

Robb Wolf is generally recognized as the foremost contemporary proponent of the Paleo Diet, as author of the New York Times best selling **The Paleo Solution—The Original Human Diet.** Robb formerly worked as a research biochemist and was a student of Professor Loren Cordain, author of **The Paleo Diet.** Robb Wolf did not discover the Paleo Diet, but his top ranked iTunes podcast, book and seminars have popularized this once-obscure way of eating.

Here are some of the specs of Wolf's biography, as found at www.robwolf.com:

"Robb has functioned as a review editor for the Journal of Nutrition and Metabolism, is co-founder of the nutrition and athletic training journal, **The Performance Menu** co-owner of **NorCal Strength & Conditioning,** one of the Men's Health "top 30 gyms in America" and he is a consultant for the Naval Special Warfare Resiliency program. He serves on the board of Directors/Advisors for: Specialty Health Inc, Paleo FX, and Paleo Magazine.

Robb is a former California State Powerlifting Champion (565 lb. Squat, 345 lb. Bench, 565 lb. Dead Lift) and a 6-0 amateur kickboxer. He coaches athletes at the highest levels of competition and consults with Olympians and world champions in MMA, motocross, rowing and triathlon. Wolf has provided seminars in nutrition and strength & conditioning to a number of entities including NASA, Naval Special Warfare, the Canadian Light Infantry and the United States Marine Corps.

Robb lives in Reno, Nevada with his wife Nicki and daughter Zoe. The following is his definition of what comprises the Paleo Diet:

"In simple terms, the Paleo Diet is built from modern foods that (to the best of our ability) emulate the foods available to our pre-agricultural ancestors: Meat, fish, fowl, vegetables, fruits, roots, tubers and nuts. On the flip-side we see an omission of grains, legumes and dairy...In simple terms, if it's not meat, fish, fowl, vegetables, fruits, roots tubers or nuts...it's a "no-go.

"In addition to food we like to consider things like sleep, stress and vitamin D levels (for a short list) as a move away from ancestral norms appears to be very important when we are concerned about performance, health and longevity." (www.robbwolf.com)

More Than a Diet

Many of those who embrace the Paleo way of life approach it as an all-encompassing lifestyle, not just a diet. Some of the non-food-related factors given consideration are sleep, exercise, relaxation and quality relationships. The goal of the Paleo approach to these is to mimic the lifestyle of pre-agricultural mankind on the premise that our caveman predecessors enjoyed a better quality of life than we do now.

Take stress, for example. Pre-agricultural humans had relatively little stress. They enjoyed long leisure hours of socializing and rest after eating a deer, bison or wild hog. Their work of hunting was intense but brief, followed by several days of eating meat.

Life in the media-saturated western civilization of the twenty-first century is characterized by unrelenting stress. Even children take their problems to bed with them, if they are allowed to text their friends, chat on snapchat or instagram, or post on Facebook. Children of earlier generations might have a terrible time with bullies at school, but at least there was a time of reprieve when they got home. Life has become an information overload that keeps our adrenalin pumping, until the adrenal glands become too worn out to pump anymore.

For the pre-agricultural human, stress was of a very different sort. Danger was not at all subtle; it came in the form of a warring tribe, or a ferocious beast. The fight-or-flight instinct of the hunter/gatherer was highly developed. People were generally at rest, or they were literally fighting for their lives. Few of us ever experience stress of this nature or degree. Every sinew was primed for action, but that action, for all of its intensity, was relatively brief.

Pre-agricultural people spent a lot of time out of doors, soaking in the vitamin D3 of the sun. Work was physical and involved lifting, stooping, running and throwing. Research of human remains has demonstrated that the human body grew significantly smaller in stature after people started growing and eating crops. We might like bread; the Lord's Prayer in the Bible even asks God to give it to us each day. But the evidence mounts continually that bread, pasta, oats, quinoa, rice—every sort of grain- - are not useful for promoting health in our bodies. Likewise, we are ill-adapted to digest legumes, like beans, as these are also crops introduced to the human diet relatively recently.

Enter the Paleo Lifestyle—and lifestyle is really what it's all about. Going Paleo is a way of life, not just a way of eating. The goal of today's Paleo is to emulate the aspects of primitive life that are beneficial for promoting health, while continuing to live within the context of modern culture. Thus, the person who is Paleo through and through lives, to the best of his or her ability, by these basic tenets:

- Eat like a caveman.
- Spend time in the sun.
- Play

- Lift heavy things
- Run in short, intense bursts.

While many great books have been written on all aspects of Paleo living, the focus of this report is mainly diet. Indeed, diet is the most foundational aspect of Paleo life, because it's healthful diet that gives us the latitude to pursue the other aspects. As goes the diet and nutrition, so goes the quality—and quantity—of life.

Low Carb, NOT No Carb

The Paleo Diet resembles the Atkins Diet and the Primal Diet in some ways, there are also important differences. While Atkins severely restricts carbohydrate intake, forbidding most fruits and vegetables, the Paleo Diet encourages eating fruits and vegetables, in moderation. There are good carbs and bad carbs; grains are bad carbs, while fruits and vegetables are good carbs. If you are counting carbohydrates, a good number to shoot for is 100 grams per day, or less. The Primal Diet is a little less strict than the Paleo regarding the consumption of dairy products.

Low Carb Flu Season

When you begin eating Paleo, your body stops producing most of its glucose from carbohydrates and begins producing it from fats and proteins. Our bodies are fully capable of making this transition, but it can take some time. During this transitional phase, many new Paleoites experience a phenomenon affectionately known as "the low carb flu."

The symptoms of this temporary discomfort include low energy and mental fogginess. If you have struggled with hypoglycemic attacks in the past, these attacks may (temporarily) become more frequent. Some people don't experience any discomfort at all, while others suffer more intensely. Overall, people who have been eating a lower carbohydrate for some time tend not to struggle as much as those who have been real carbohydrate addicts. However, this isn't a hard and fast rule. In every case, however, the low carb flu is temporary, if you stick it out and don't give in to the temptation to go back to eating grains and other refined carbohydrates. Studies have shown the initial disadvantages of low carb eating are erased after this window of time.

For many people, symptoms of the low carb flu tend to disappear in between one to three weeks. Occasionally, the discomfort might last up to one month. What's going on in your body, according to Mark Sisson, is that you are actually shifting metabolic related gene expression, increasing fat oxidation pathways, and decreasing fat storage pathways.

"Within a few weeks, your body becomes fairly efficient at converting protein and fat for the liver's glycogen stores, which provide all the glucose we need for the brain, red blood cells, muscles, etcetera, under regular circumstances" (Mark Sisson, Mark's Daily Apple).

The main thing to remember is that although you feel as though you are hurting your body by not continuing to fill it with glucose, you are actually doing your brain a big favor. Recent evidence suggests that Alzheimer's Disease is a kind of "type 3" diabetes, a disease related to insulin resistance.

Also keep in mind that people who are transitioning to low carb eating can actually shortchange their physical needs when they don't eat enough fat, or when they pursue high intensity exercise routines. You can help yourself by easing up on your carb restriction a little bit by adding 25 grams or so. Listen to your body; if it tells you that you should eat an extra serving of vegetables with dinner (for added carbohydrates), go ahead and do it. Don't be surprised if you find you need a little extra sleep. Drinking green tea at the right time might also help you get through the rough time. The temporary setback of the low carb flu is as nothing, compared to the benefits once you have made the transition.

Get Ready to Eat Delicious Food

Once you realize how much sumptuous food is available to you on the Paleo Diet, you won't even miss the grains and legumes you used to eat. New converts to Paleo often make the mistake of trying to substitute grain-free alternatives for the simple carbohydrates they are used to. This subtle trap can undermine your success, and it makes you feel as though you are missing out.

Face it: there is no acceptable substitute for a fresh, hot piece of bread, straight from the oven. "Bread" made with almond or coconut meal might appeal to you, but it also might feel like a cruel joke.

The Importance of Eating Grass-Fed Beef, Organic Chicken, Free Range Eggs, and Wild Caught Fish

Remember that essentially, when you eat an animal or animal by-product, you are eating what the animal you are eating ate. (You might have to read that last sentence a few times to wrap your mind around it.)

If you are avoiding grains in your diet, you also need to avoid eating animals that ate grains. Farm raised fish, for example, is fed grain pellets. So if you eat farm raised tilapia, you are eating second hand grains. The same goes for beef and chicken. Grain fed beef and chicken pass those grains along to you when you eat them.

Commercially raised, grain fed beef is pumped full of hormones to stimulate faster growth. When you eat this beef, keep in mind that you are also eating the hormones. Commercially produced chickens are fed antibiotics, as well as hormones and grains. It's hard to even conceive of how many unhealthy things you consume with every bite of a mass-produced bird!

A Few Recipes to Get You Started

The humble little selection of recipes presented here is by no means a complete cookbook. There are many terrific Paleo cookbooks on the market; my recipe collection doesn't even fall into the category of cookbook! The purpose of my sharing these recipes with you is to give you an idea of what sorts of things I eat and enjoy on a limited budget. I hope that these recipes will convey to you that eating Paleo doesn't have to be complicated. You might even laugh at how ridiculously simple it is to eat like a king!

When I look back at all of the complicated steps I used to follow to prepare carbohydrate, chemical laden casseroles, the truth is underscored for manyfold that simple really **is** better!

Baked, Spiced Veal

1 large cut of veal
butter
minced garlic
sea salt
curry powder
parsley flakes
powdered ginger
paprika
black pepper

Preheat oven to 375.

Melt butter in skillet over medium low heat. Turn heat up to medium high, and add veal. Sear for about one minute per side to seal in juices. Remove from stove.

Transfer veal to a baking dish. Sprinkle both sides with all of the herbs and spices.

Bake, uncovered, for about 40 minutes, or until done to your liking.

Paleo Chik-Fil-A

1 pound (500 g) of chicken breasts, cut into large chunks

1/3 cup dill pickle juice

1 egg, beaten
1 Tablespoon coconut milk
1 Tablespoon coconut flour
1 Tablespoon arrowroot flour
1/2 Tablespoon paprika (sweet or smoked)
1/2 teaspoon sea salt
1/2 teaspoon black pepper
1/2 teaspoon onion powder
1/4 teaspoon garlic powder
Coconut oil for frying

Cut the chicken breast into large chunks, and put it in a zip top plastic bag. Pour the pickle juice into the bag. Let it marinate in the refrigerator for at least 2 hours. (I kept it in overnight).

After it's done marinating, pour the pickle juice out of the bag.

In a small bowl, mix the beaten egg and coconut milk. Pour that into the bag and let it sit for about 10 minutes while you prepare the spice mix.

In another small bowl, mix the coconut flour, arrowroot flour, smoked paprika, salt, pepper, onion power and garlic powder.

Open the bag and drain out as much egg/coconut milk as you can. It doesn't have to be 100% dry because you want something for the spice mix to stick to.

Pour the spice mix into the bag, close the top, and really massage it into the chicken. This may take a minute or two but you want all the pieces to be evenly coated.

In a large skillet over medium-high, heat a few tablespoons of coconut oil until the oil is very hot. Add a single layer of chicken (being careful not to crowd it) to the pan and fry on each side for about 3 minutes or until it's completely cooked through. It took me two batches to cook one pound of chicken.

(from www.stupideasypaleo.com)

Marinated, Grilled Salmon Filets

2 large, wild-caught salmon filets
vinaigrette

<u>To Prepare Vinaigrette</u>
6 tablespoons extra virgin olive oil
2 tablespoons balsamic vinaigrette
¼ teaspoon brown mustard
dash of sea salt
grinding of fresh, black pepper

Add all vinaigrette ingredients to a large ziplock freezer bag; seal bag and shake until thoroughly emulsified.

Place salmon filets in the bag. Seal and marinate in the refrigerator for at least 4 hours. Turn the bag once during this time, if you can, to ensure uniform marination.

Heat grill on medium low. Put salmon on grill, and cover.

Grill for 4 minutes on each side, or until fish flakes easily with a fork.

Great with Greek Salad!

Sausage Stir-Fry Breakfast

1 tsp coconut oil

½ yellow onion, diced

½ lb. Sausages (nitrate/nitrite free), sliced

4 cups of spinach or other greens

Heat a skillet over medium heat, and add coconut oil when hot.

Add diced onions and sauté until slightly translucent.

Add sausage and cook until browned, tossing frequently.

Add greens, reduce heat to medium-low, and cover.

Serve when the greens are wilted and soft (about 5 minutes).

(from www.paleoplan.com)

Fruit Salad with Cinnamon

1 orange, peeled and diced

1 apple, diced

1/2 cup pecans or walnuts, chopped (optional)

1/2 tsp cinnamon

Place the fruit into bowls.

Sprinkle with chopped nuts (optional) and/or cinnamon.

Add coconut milk for more calories, if desired.

(from www.paleoplan.com)

Fried Eggs

½ lb. Bacon
3 Eggs

Cook bacon in a skillet. Place on a paper towel to drain.

Pour off all but 1 tablespoon bacon grease, and re-heat skillet to medium low.

Carefully break open eggs, and slide them into the skillet.

Cover skillet to steam eggs.

If you like eggs over-easy, they should be ready to flip in about three minutes.

Eat with bacon!

Banana Smoothie

Almond or coconut milk
Raw egg
Ripe banana
¼ teaspoon Stevia extract
1 scoop whey protein powder
Pinch Nutmeg

Blend egg and liquid in a blender.

Break banana into small chunks and add to liquid, along with stevia and nutmeg. Blend.

Add protein, and blend once more.

Serves 2.

Coconut Braised Parsnips

4 parsnips, chopped into rings
2 tablespoons extra virgin coconut oil
ground cinnamon, ginger and nutmeg
dash of salt

Melt the coconut oil in a skillet on medium heat. Add the parsnips, and stir until coated with oil. Cover and fry for ten minutes, stirring occasionally. Add cinnamon, ginger and nutmeg to taste. Toss with a dash of salt, and serve hot.

Serves four.

Mashed Sweet Potato Divinity

2 sweet potatoes, chopped or sliced
3 tablespoons almond milk
3 tablespoons unsalted butter
cinnamon
pure vanilla extract
stevia extract
salt

Put chopped sweet potatoes into a microwaveable ceramic dish with a lid. Add almond milk and slices of butter. Cover dish, and microwave for 13 minutes. Mash cooked sweet potatoes with a fork, and add a dash of vanilla extract for extra flavor and moisture. Add a pinch of stevia and salt. Sprinkle liberally with cinnamon, and mix thoroughly.

This side dish makes a fabulous accompaniment to a beef main course!

Serves 3.

Sautéed Portabella Mushrooms

16 ounce container of sliced Portabella mushrooms
3 tablespoons unsalted butter
shot of garlic salt

Melt butter over low heat. Add mushrooms, and cook gradually over low to medium heat for approximately 7 minutes. Mushrooms are done when they are soft and brown, but not mushy. Toss with garlic salt and serve hot.

Serves 4.

Eggplant with Onions and Peppers

1 medium eggplant, chopped into cubes
1 medium red, orange and yellow pepper (3 peppers total), sliced
1 medium chopped sweet onion
2 tablespoons extra virgin olive oil
basil
rosemary
oregano
salt
pepper
organic vegetable stock

Heat olive oil in a large skillet over medium high heat. Add onions and peppers; turn heat down to medium and sautee for 3 minutes. Add cubed eggplant, and toss to coat. Sprinkle with spices, herbs, and a liberal shot of vegetable stock. Cover skillet, and cook on low until eggplant is cooked through, about 5 minutes.

Take care not to overcook. The eggplant should no longer be white and springy. It should be very soft, but not mushy.

Serves 4.

Wilted Lemon Spinach

Large bag of pre-washed baby spinach leaves
2-3 tablespoons butter
juice of ¼ lemon
coarse sea salt, to taste

Melt butter over low heat. Add spinach leaves, and increase heat to medium.

Raw spinach leaves have a lot of volume, so you will have to keep pushing them down into the skillet for the first few minutes of cooking!

Cover skillet; turn heat down to low. Keep a close eye on the skillet, and toss leaves at regular intervals.

The spinach is ready to eat when the leaves are wilted and coated with butter, but still bright green.

Squeeze lemon juice over the top, and sprinkle with sea salt. Toss one more time.

Serves 4.

Baked Zucchini

3 large zucchini, sliced diagonally
olive oil
pastry or kitchen utility brush
coarse sea salt
freshly ground pepper

Preheat oven to 275 degrees. Brush sliced zucchini with olive oil, and place on an ungreased cookie sheet. Sprinkle zucchini with sea salt and ground pepper from grinder. Bake for 10 minutes; turn zucchini slices over with tongs. Brush again with olive oil, and repeat salt and pepper. Bake for 10 more minutes, and serve.

Serves 4.

Baked Chicken Thighs

Six large chicken thighs with skin on
Extra virgin olive oil
Utility brush
Coarse sea salt
Freshly ground pepper

Preheat oven to 275 degrees. Place chicken thighs into a large casserole dish, skin up. Brush skin with olive oil; sprinkle with salt and a scant grinding of pepper.

Bake, uncovered, for one hour, or until skin is crispy and golden brown.

Serves 6.

The Easiest Avocado Snack Ever

Avocado
Coarse sea salt
Freshly ground black pepper

The secret to eating a perfect avocado is knowing when it is perfectly ready to cut. The avocado should yield *just slightly* to pressure between your thumb and forefinger. If the fruit is very soft, make guacamole. If it is hard as a rock, wait a couple of days before cutting it.

When the avocado is ready, cut it in half vertically, using a sharp knife. Separate the two halves using gentle pressure. Remove the pit with a spoon.

Sprinkle with salt and pepper. Eat right out of the shell, scooping the meat out with a spoon.

If you are on the go and don't have salt and pepper with you, this makes a great snack without any seasoning at all!

Frozen Fruit "Sherbet"

Bagged frozen fruit of your choice from the frozen foods section of your market
  (I like the strawberry/pineapple/mango/peach combo best)
Smattering of stevia powder

Pour a generous serving of frozen fruit into a bowl. Allow to thaw at room temperature for five minutes. Sprinkle with stevia.

If you are in a hurry for dessert, you can thaw the fruit in the microwave for 35 seconds before sprinkling with stevia.

The consistency of this all-natural confection will be like that of a popsicle.
Mmmm—Enjoy!

Grilled Ribeye Steak

Grass-fed ribeye steaks, ½ inch thick
Coarse sea salt
Freshly ground pepper

Preheat grill on high. Turn heat down slightly, and toss on steaks. Sere slightly on both slides to retain juices. Grill steaks and flip them over, cooking until they have reached your desired degree of doneness.

Medium steaks will require about 4 minutes of cooking on the first side and 3 minutes on the second.

Well-done steaks (no pink) will require about 5 minutes per side.

With grass-fed steak, you can feel free to eat and enjoy the fat, which makes the meat more tender and flavorful.

Marinated, Grilled Chicken Breasts

Extra virgin olive oil
Balsamic vinegar
Italian herbs, such as oregano, thyme and basil
Dash of vegetable stock
Salt and pepper, to taste
4 large boneless, skinless organic chicken breasts

In the morning, prepare marinade in a large ziplock bag as follows:
- two tablespoons balsamic vinegar
- six tablespoons extra virgin olive oil
- dash of vegetable stock
- Italian herbs
- Salt and pepper

Place the chicken breasts in the bag, and squeeze out the air before sealing. Marinate in the refrigerator for at least 4 hours, turning the bag over after 2 hours.

Preheat grill on high. Turn down heat to somewhere between low and medium, and toss on chicken breasts.

Grill breasts for about 7 minutes on each side. When done, put grilled chicken into a casserole dish and cover with reserved marinade for extra tenderness and flavor.

The combination of marination, low grilling temperature, and coating of reserved marinade makes this chicken exceptionally tender and juicy! Serves 4.

Latvian Salad

Six large Roma tomatoes at the peak of ripeness
One cucumber, peeled
Organic mayonnaise
Salt

Mince cucumber into fine bits. Chop tomatoes into small pieces. Mix in a medium bowl with 1/4-1/2 cup organic mayonnaise, depending on how creamy you want the salad to be. Salt to taste.

This extremely simple salad is typically eaten as outdoor picnic fare during the summertime in Eastern Europe.

Bacon-Laced Frittata

Bacon
6 ounce bag of frozen onion and pepper medley (from vegetable section in store)
6 large eggs
Salt and pepper, to taste

Cook bacon in a large skillet until crispy. Make sure that you cook enough that you still have 4 slices left, after you have eaten all you want!

Pour off most of the bacon grease, but leave about a tablespoonful in the skillet.

Turn heat on stovetop to medium, and sautee the frozen onions and peppers in the bacon grease.

Break and scramble the eggs in a large mixing bowl.

Distribute the onions and peppers evenly throughout the skillet.

Pour the scrambled egg mixture over the top of the vegetables.

Cover the skillet, and let the eggs set while cooking on medium heat.

It is optional to flip the frittata in the pan, using two spatulas. Sometimes this works out great; sometimes, not. The golden brown top does look yummy, when you succeed.

Flip from the skillet to a serving platter. Cut into slices, and serve.
Great with salsa!

Apple with Almond Butter

One big, beautiful, juicy apple
Knife or apple slicer
Jar of the best almond butter you can afford
Plate
Spoon

Cut or slice your apple, and put the slices on the plate. Open your jar of almond butter, and spoon out a generous dollop to put on the plate beside the apple slices. Spoon almond butter onto each slice. You can double-spoon, if you want; it's your apple.

(The plate is optional, but it feels good to be genteel, even when one is eating like a caveman.)

Pepitas and Raisins

½ cup raw pumpkin seeds
¼ cup raisins

Mix pumpkin seeds thoroughly with raisins; keep the proportion of pumpkin seeds: raisins approximately 2:1, so that you don't unduly elevate your blood sugar with the sweet raisins. The fat and protein in the pumpkin seeds slow down the absorption of the natural sugar from the raisins. Crunchiness and chewiness are juxtaposed, making for a tasty mix of consistencies.

Almond Brothers Smoothie

Unsweetened vanilla almond milk
One ripe banana
2 tablespoons almond butter
1 scoop plain whey protein powder mix
blender

Put the almond milk into a blender first. Then add the other ingredients, and blend on a high setting until frothy.

If your whey protein powder is sweetened with stevia, you won't need any additional sweetener. However, if not, you might want to add a squeeze of agave nectar or a pinch of ground stevia.

If you really want to get yourself jazzed, in a protein sort of way, add a raw egg—or two. Guaranteed, you won't get hungry again for several hours after drinking this bad boy.

Greek Salad

1 tablespoon extra virgin olive oil
1 lb. boneless, skinless chicken tenders
4 roma tomatoes
1 medium cucumber
feta cheese
pitted kalamata olives
bag of spring mix greens

Sautee the chicken tenders in the olive oil, turning until thoroughly cooked throughout.

Chop tomatoes and cucumber.

Combine ½ of the bag of greens, tomato, cucumber, along with kalamata olives and feta cheese, to taste.

Top with chicken tenders. You can chop these to make them extend further.

Toss with vinaigrette dressing.

<u>Vinaigrette Dressing</u>

6 tablespoons extra virgin olive oil
2 tablespoons balsamic vinegar
dash of sea salt
grinding of fresh black pepper
splash of water, vegetable or chicken stock

Shake all ingredients in a jar to combine. Makes enough dressing for one large salad.

Tips For Making It On the Paleo Diet

As someone who has successfully made the transition to the Paleo way of eating, I have some tips to share with those who are just starting their Paleo journeys. These suggestions are all things that helped me. I don't guarantee that they will help you, but I hope so. These tips are presented in no particular order.

- Read **The Paleo Solution** by Robb Wolfe and **The Primal Revolution** by Mark Sisson. Each of these authors has his own distinct style and point of view, but they agree on most major points.

- Join a local Paleo group, if there is one near you. If not, there are many support networks and forums online. I found www.marksdailyapple.com to be particularly helpful.

- Give away the food you have in your home which you no longer want to eat. Being able to choose your way of eating is a luxury not shared by everyone. Your local food bank would probably love to have the canned, boxed or otherwise processed food items that you no longer want. Someone who would otherwise not eat can make a meal of them.

- Get comfortable with telling people that your body doesn't tolerate grains, legumes or dairy foods well. People who don't know you well probably won't ask too many questions. If anyone raises an eyebrow, simply explain that you have recently discovered these food intolerances, and that you are adjusting your diet accordingly. Trying to convince anyone else that they should go on the Paleo Diet, too, is a waste of breath. Wait until they see your results; then they will beg you to tell them how you did it!

- Familiarize yourself with stores and farms where you can obtain your food. Not every food market carries grass fed beef or bison, for example. You might find a local organic farmer who will sell you half or a quarter of a cow. You also may be able to buy free range eggs more cheaply from an individual than from an organic grocery store.

- Be realistic about what you can afford. Make a list of your priorities for expensive items, and keep your feet on the ground when you shop. It can be fun and exciting to try higher quality foods. However, shopping beyond your means is a sure way to shipwreck your efforts.

- Remember that Paleo is not so much a diet as a way of eating. This isn't something that you'll be doing for a little while; it's a whole lifestyle change. Be honest with yourself about whether or not the transition to Paleo is worth the cost to you. People normally don't make major lifestyle changes until the pain of maintaining the *status quo* is greater than the perceived pain of making a switch.

- Prepare yourself for at least a couple of rough weeks, as your body adjusts to not having its daily carbohydrate fix. When you are really feeling lousy, it is especially important to have external support.

- If your body craves something that is allowed on the Paleo Diet, indulge your craving, at least to a moderate degree. Cravings are often our body's way of telling us what they need. However, remember that your carbohydrate cravings stem from an unhealthy addiction. If you are craving bacon, eat bacon (as I did). If you are craving steak, eat steak (if you can). An avocado craving isn't a weird fetish; it might be the beginning of a beautiful relationship!

- Think ahead. This skill takes time to establish, but it is essential to your success at the Paleo way. Processed foods are not only less expensive than whole, organic foods, they are also faster to prepare. When you are eating Paleo, you have to think about what you are going to have for dinner before 4:30 p.m.! In fact, you actually need to plan your dinner in the morning, at the latest. If you will be eating meat that is currently frozen, remember to thaw it out. If you want to have spinach salad, make sure that you have spinach in the fridge, or make a note to pick some up.

- Remember that you will invariably eat the food that you keep in your house. If you want to eat pumpkin seeds and raisins, or celery with almond butter, for a snack, make sure that you buy them instead of Ritz crackers.

- Find a Paleo-friendly food that you particularly love, and keep some of it on hand. When the going gets tough, the tough eat dark chocolate. Or frozen cherries. Or whatever it is that you really dig. This is especially important if you live in a household where some members (your children, for example) aren't completely into the "Paleo thing." If your kids are having spaghetti, and spaghetti used to be your favorite food, be prepared to treat yourself to something else special.

- Take some food with you when you are going out for a couple of hours. You will probably soon find that you can go much longer between meals than you used to. However, if you have an avocado and some trail mix in your lunchbox, and you take your lunchbox with you, you are much less likely to grab a bag of potato chips at the gas station.

- Buy a lunchbox!

- If you are caught hungry and don't have food on hand, buy a snack at a grocery store, instead of a fast food restaurant.

- Take on one new challenge at a time. The month you are transitioning from processed food to Paleo is not the time to start a rigorous new exercise program!

- If you can afford it, treat yourself to a new pair of jeans when your old ones get too big!

- Learn how to accept compliments graciously. When someone tells you that you look fantastic, a simple "thank you" is all that is needed.

- If you find yourself sabotaging your eating goals, look for the secondary payoff you could be getting by doing so. For example, if you are known throughout your whole family for making great Swedish pancakes, you might sabotage your Paleo eating efforts by cooking—and eating—a monster breakfast with Swedish pancakes. At that moment, the pleasure you get from your identity as the world's best maker of Swedish pancakes is greater than your resolve not to eat flour.

- Get comfortable with being uncomfortable. For a little while, at least. For many people, the Paleo Diet is shipwrecked on the iceberg of New, Strange and Different. Making big changes is hard. The secondary gain that might tempt you most is familiarity. We are all creatures of habit, and familiarity is synonymous with comfort. Bear in mind, however, that comfort is highly overrated.

- You know what your goals are. Keep them in view. However, don't get fixated on the end result, or you can become discouraged by the fact that you're not there yet. Sometimes, the best thing to focus on is simply doing the next right thing. If you keep on doing the next right thing, day after day, the long-term result you want will take care of itself.

- Drink plenty of water. If you can't afford filtered water, which is better? Tap water or a diet Coke? For most people reading this report, the tap water would be the better choice.

- To afford Paleo sometimes choosing the lesser of two evils. I sometimes eat slim jims when I am hungry all of a sudden. They are filled with chemicals and aren't healthy choice, by any means. But my cholesterol is great, and I still wear a size 4 jeans.

- Nut butters are better than peanut butter, because peanuts are a legume. But common sense tells you that the action of peanut butter on the body is similar to that of other nut butters. If you can't afford a $17 jar of raw almond butter, don't stress about it. Buy the roasted almond butter. If you can't afford that, buy the all natural peanut butter. If you can't afford that, a jar of Jif is better than a piece of cake. Use your brain.

- If you are out and you get hungry, go to a supermarket instead of a fast food restaurant. You can get fruit, an avocado, a hunk of meat from the deli, they always have plastic cutlery that they give you for free. It ends up being cheaper than fast food, and you don't have to pay the price of bruising your conscience, either.

Paleo Diet Food List

This comprehensive list contains Paleo Diet meats, vegetables, fruits, nuts, seeds and desserts.

Paleo Diet Meats

- Poultry
- Turkey
- Chicken Breast
- Pork Tenderloin
- Pork Chops
- Steak
- Bacon
- Pork chops
- Ground Beef
- Grass Fed Beef
- Chicken Thigh
- Chicken Leg
- Chicken Wings
- Lamb rack
- Shrimp
- Lobster
- Clams
- Salmon
- Venison Steaks
- Buffalo
- New York Steak
- Chops
- Rabbit
- Goat
- Bear

Paleo Diet Eggs

- Duck
- Chicken
- Goose

Paleo Diet Vegetables

Almost all vegetables foods are on the Paleo Diet. However, the starchy ones should be consumed in moderation. Vegetables with a high starch content, like potatoes, and squashes, tend to have low nutritional value in comparison to the amount of starches/carbs/sugars they contain. While they're not bad for you, be careful not to overdo them.

- Asparagus
- Avocado
- Artichoke hearts
- Brussels sprouts
- Carrots
- Spinach
- Celery
- Broccoli
- Zucchini
- Cabbage
- Peppers (All Kinds)
- Cauliflower
- Parsley
- Eggplant
- Green Onions
- Butternut Squash*
- Acorn Squash*
- Yam*
- Sweet Potato*
- Beets

These starchy foods are great for energy replacement for Paleo diet athletes who spend long periods of time exercising and need some of the starchier foods on the Paleo diet to sustain their energy levels. As long as you're training, you'll find these are great sources of energy replacements, especially post- workout. However, if you're trying to lose weight on the Paleo diet, you'll want to limit the quantities of these that you're eating.

Paleo Diet Fruits**

Paleo diet fruits are not only delicious, they're great for you. Fruits, however, even Paleo-approved ones, contain large amounts of fructose which – while much better than HFCS (high-fructose corn syrup) – is still sugar. If you're looking to lose weight on the Paleo diet, you'll want to cut back on the fruit intake and focus more on vegetables. Otherwise, feel free to have 1-3 servings of fruit a day.

- Apple

- Avocado
- Blackberries
- Papaya
- Peaches
- Plums
- Mango
- Lychee
- Blueberries
- Grapes
- Lemon
- Strawberries
- Watermelon
- Pineapple Guava
- Lime
- Raspberries
- Cantaloupe
- Tangerine
- Figs
- Oranges
- Bananas*

*These starchy foods are great for energy replacement for Paleo diet athletes
who spend long periods of time exercising and need some of the starchier foods on the Paleo diet
to sustain their energy levels. As long as you're training, you'll find these are great sources of energy
replacements, especially post- workout. However, if you're trying to lose weight on the Paleo diet,
you'll want to limit the quantities of these that you're eating.*

**Eat high-sugar fruits and vegetables in moderation.*

Paleo Diet Oils/Fats

Eat Good Fats!

Understand that not all fat is bad! Fat creates *satiety*, or a feeling of being full, which prevents you from overeating. Fat also slows down the absorption of carbohydrates as they are converted to sugar in the body. This helps maintain healthy blood sugar levels, as your blood sugar rises more slowly in the presence of fat.

When blood sugar plateaus after a meal containing fat, it stays on that nice, level plateau for several hours, before it gradually starts to descend, and you feel hungry again. Natural oils and fats are your body's preferred way of creating energy so it's best to give your body what it's asking for! The following are some of the best types of Paleo oils and fats that you can give your body if you're in need of some additional sustained energy.

- Coconut oil
- Olive oil
- Macadamia Oil
- Avocado Oil
- Grass fed Butter

Foods labeled "fat free" are usually highly processed, contain a lot of chemicals, and almost invariably contain high fructose corn syrup.

Paleo Diet Nuts

Nuts are decidedly Paleo. Be careful, as cashews and peanuts are high in fat and for some reason, It's incredibly easy to eat an entire jar in one sitting. If you're trying to lose weight, limit the amount of nuts you're consuming.

- Almonds
- Cashews
- Hazelnuts
- Pecans
- Pine Nuts
- Pumpkin Seeds
- Sunflower Seeds
- Macadamia Nuts
- Walnuts

Sweeteners

- monk fruit
- agave
- stevia (This has no calories)
- honey
- maple syrup

Although all of these sweeteners are allowed on the Paleo Diet, you may soon find that you don't have the same need you used to have to sweeten everything. Eating Paleo, you will start taste the natural sweetness that you never noticed before, in fruits, and even in vegetables An orange becomes something truly glorious.

Foods Not Allowed on The Paleo Diet

These foods are not allowed on the Paleo Diet:

Dairy

What About Dairy?

Whether or not to completely avoid dairy products is a controversial subject in the Paleo world. Milk is very glycogenic; this just means that it contains a lot of sugar. Many, if not most, adults become increasingly lactose intolerant as they age, so consuming dairy products, especially drinking milk, can cause belching, bloating and/or flatulence. In full-blown lactose intolerance, eating dairy may result in diarrhea.

This being said, Paleo-types who aren't quite so strict (leaning more toward the Primal diet) do, on occasion, consume a little dairy. Butter, heavy whipping cream, Greek yogurt, and hard cheeses tend not to cause digestive problems to the degree caused by other forms of dairy.

To find out the best scenario for you, go on a dairy elimination diet. Cut out dairy completely for 30 days. Then, slowly re-introduce one dairy product into your diet, and observe the consequences, if any, to your feeling of physical well-being. It is best to test only one dairy product at a time, so that you can know what is causing what.

If you opt to eliminate dairy from your diet, these foods need to go:

- Butter
- Cheese
- Cottage Cheese
- Non fat dairy creamer
- Skim milk
- 2% milk
- Whole milk (sometimes)
- Dairy spreads
- Cream cheese
- Powdered milk

- Yogurt
- Pudding
- Frozen Yogurt
- Ice Milk
- Low fat milk
- Ice cream

Soft drinks

If, occasionally, you can't live without a soda, drink a regular one, rather than a diet soda. Diet sodas actually promote weight gain, and the artificial sweeteners they contain are nothing short of poisonous.

Try to find soda made with real cane sugar, instead of high fructose corn syrup.

Also, most health food stores carry sodas that are sweetened with stevia extract. These are a good option for a once-in-a-while treat.

Fruit Juices--These should be avoided, as they are extremely high in sugar.

- Apple Juice
- Orange Juice
- Grape Juice
- Strawberry Juice
- Chinola Juice
- Starfruit Juice
- Mango Juice

Grains

Tip: Don't waste time or money trying to make your diet mimic a diet with grains. Just accept that you don't eat those anymore, and go on with life, fully enjoying the things that you can and do eat.

I tell people that I am allergic to grains. Eating grains causes me to be sluggish, unable to concentrate, irritable, have headaches, fat, flatulent. If that isn't allergy, I don't know what allergy is. Telling people that you are allergic to grains, or that your body can't tolerate them, saves you from a lot of trouble trying to explain why you eat the way you do.

Maybe smart people will put two and two together and figure out that that's why you look so darn good!

My experiment making pancakes with almond meal. I thought I had to replace the bread-like foods I used to eat. What I eventually found was that I didn't miss those foods at all:

- Cereals
- Bread
- English Muffin
- Toast
- Sandwiches
- Crackers of any kind
- Oatmeal
- Cream of Wheat
- Corn
- Wheat of any kind, including sprouted
- Pasta
- Rice Barley
- Quinoa
- Any other grain

Simple carbohydrates turn your body into a blood sugar roller coaster ride. The body becomes resistant to the action of the insulin produced by your pancreas, and you actually become a fat manufacturing machine. By contrast, Paleo dieters are fat burning machines.

For a complete scientific information of insulin resistance, please refer to **The Paleo Solution** by Robb Wolf.

Legumes

- Peanuts
- Peanut butter

All beans, including:

- Black Beans
- Broad Beans
- Fava Beans
- Garbanzo Beans
- Horse Beans
- Kidney Beans
- Lima Beans
- Mung Beans
- Adzuki Beans
- Navy Beans

- Pinto Beans
- Red Beans
- Green Beans
- String Beans
- White Beans

Peas

- Black Eyed Peas
- Chickpeas
- Snowpeas
- Sugar snap peas
- Miso
- Lentils
- Lupins
- Mesquite
- Soybeans
- All soybean products and derivatives
- Tofu

Bad Fats

- Canola oil
- Peanut oil
- Anything that calls itself "vegetable oil"
- Margarine

Miscellaneous

Fatty Meats
Spam
Hot Dogs
Other low-quality meats
Salty Foods
Starchy Vegetables

<u>**Sweets**</u>

Remember the 80/20 rule. If you completely forbid yourself to ever eat sugar, you will probably rebel against your own edict and eat too much of it.

Plan, instead, to have a little sweet treat now and then. Half a bar of dark chocolate makes a great dessert. I eat chocolate almost every day, and I don't have either weight or blood sugar problems because of it. But I don't eat a whole bar.

Odds and Ends:

Miscellaneous Aspects of Paleo Living

The Danger of Excessive Exercise

A diet that includes grains automatically promotes insulin resistance, which, in turn, promotes weight gain. Thus, if your typical breakfast consists of a bagel, toast, oatmeal or cereal and juice, you will find it hard to lose weight, even if you exercise daily.

Here is a typical scenario: a 35 year old woman is 5'5" and weighs 150 pounds. She desperately wants to take of 25 pounds, so she jogs three miles, five days per week. She thinks to herself that ironically, she is the healthiest overweight person she knows. No matter how she punishes her body, she doesn't lose an ounce.

She eats fat free foods, drinks diet sodas, and makes sure that all of her meats are lean. Why is she stuck in this frustrating pattern? Why does she work so hard, yet get so little in return?

The answer is twofold. First of all, the grains in her diet set her up for insulin resistance that make it almost impossible to lose weight. Secondly, her mode of exercise is long, slow cardiovascular workout.

This type of exercise, although popular in our culture, is limited in its usefulness for training.

Short bursts of intense exercise, followed by short periods of rest, are called **intervals**. Interval training is the most effective method of burning fat. Your body burns stored fat, not just while you are exercising, but up to 24 hours afterward. Long, slow cardio, on the other hand, burns fat, but only during the period of exercise. This type of training is much harder on the joints than interval training. But so many people gravitate towards it anyway, because of the myth that the more painful the exercise, the better it is for the body. Fact facts: you are beating your body up, and you still aren't getting the results you want.

Interval training, or running for brief, intense bursts with a short recovery time in between, is very intense and is, of course, tiring. But if you want to see lasting results in your workouts, cut the grains out of your diet, and give interval training and weight lifting a try. You will be pleasantly surprised to find out that the best, most effective workouts aren't necessarily the ones that beat your body the most.

When you eat Paleo, you will lose weight. Then exercise becomes easier. Losing weight is 80% diet and 20% exercise. Exercise is important, but diet is more essential. When you get the diet part down, the exercise part becomes a lot easier on its own. Think of carrying 50 pound weights up the stairs, every time you walk up the steps. Then think of bounding up those same steps without the 50 pounds. In which scenario are you more likely to want to take the stairs?

A Matter of Priorities

Most of us have a limited amount of discretionary income, so setting priorities about spending it is essential. The more income you have, the less painful eating Paleo will be to your pocketbook. If your income isn't unlimited, you will have to put "good food" high on your list of priorities for spending. This might mean that something else has to go.

But wait a minute—let's think this thing through. You could spend your money on good food, wearing an old pair of skinny jeans and a t-shirt, looking and feeling great. Or you could eat cheap, processed food, wearing an outfit that obviously cost a lot, looking and feeling bloated and chubby. Which scenario do you prefer? I thought so.

Avoiding Perfectionism Will Help You Succeed!

One of the quickest ways to kill your success at any endeavor is to become a slave to perfection. The pursuit of perfection can quickly result in paralysis that prevents you from doing anything. It is so important for us to be gentle with ourselves and learn how to be satisfied with "good enough!"

Mark Sisson, who pioneered the Primal Diet offshoot of Paleo, advocates the 80/20 rule: eat according to your diet 80% of the time, and don't sweat the other 20%. Cut yourself some slack.

If you are independently wealthy and have nothing but free time, you might find it possible to eat 100% Paleo, 100% of the time. For the rest of us, however, unavoidable constraints of time and resources make perfection an unattainable dream.

For some people, the inability to achieve perfection becomes an excuse not to try at all. I personally know someone who lived in a homeless shelter for almost three months and was able to maintain a reasonable Paleo diet. If she did it under those circumstances, you can, too. You just have to use common sense.

It would be superb if we could all afford only grass-fed beef, organic fruits and vegetables, wild-caught fish and cage-free, antibiotic-free chicken and eggs all of the time. If you are one of the fortunate few who has access to these foods every day that is really great. But if not, use your head. Is it better to eat a grain-fed, all-beef patty or a Snickers bar? Is it better to have an omelet made with regular, commercial eggs for breakfast, or a jelly donut?

If you can't do Paleo perfectly, do the best you can. You will see and feel results, and your body will thank you. I don't know this for a fact, but my guess is that many people never get started eating Paleo, because they tell themselves they can't afford it. Don't let the elusive pursuit of perfection prevent you from doing the best you can. If, in the end, you are afraid of the discomfort you will experience while your body adjusts to the Paleo way of eating, be honest with yourself. Failing to try because you can't be perfect is never acceptable.

Be Selective When Buying Organic

One way of cutting costs is to buy organic fruits and vegetables only when it really counts. Fruits with thin skins, like berries, grapes and apples, absorb pesticides easily. Buying organic is important where these items are concerned. Other fruits that should be organic are kiwi, plums, mangoes, and peaches.

However eating only organic oranges, bananas or pineapples is less crucial, because the peels or rinds of these fruits are thick. Pesticides probably won't penetrate to a meaningful degree. Likewise, watermelon, honeydew, and cantaloupe won't be tainted by pesticides because of their thick rinds.

My Story

For several decades, I was a sluggish, lethargic, somewhat overweight woman who was plagued with low blood sugar attacks on an almost-daily basis. I never thought much about my lack of energy; that was just "me." I had always been that way, and I assumed that I always would be.

My diet was not overly filled with grains or other refined carbohydrates, but I ate some of these every day. When I left the house, especially in the afternoon, I was careful to carry a snack. If I didn't have something to eat around 4:00 in the afternoon, I paid dearly for the omission—and so did my family, who got the brunt of my wild, tearful emotional low blood sugar outbursts. I had been diagnosed with insulin resistance, and I was on the border of becoming a Type II diabetic.

My husband Bill struggled, as I did, to maintain his desired weight. It seemed as though we just couldn't look good naked, even though we both exercised frequently! One day, he told me that he was desperate enough to try anything—even the Paleo Diet.

"What's the Paleo Diet?" was my response. He said he didn't know for sure, but some of his colleagues were on it, and they had lost a lot of weight. I recalled that one of those co-workers had visited us a few months before. Two things in particular had struck me about this woman: my dogs loved her, and she radiated good health and fitness. Her skin glowed, she was toned, and there wasn't an ounce of extra fat anywhere on her body. She had extolled the virtues of the Paleo Diet during that visit. Maybe it was time for us to give it a try. "I'll do it for Bill," I thought. "Poor Bill. Maybe it will help him. I'll go on this diet with him, just to give him encouragement."

That night, I did some research online to find out exactly what the Paleo Diet entailed. I read that it was a grain-free, dairy-free, legume free diet that focused on eating mainly meat, poultry, fish, fruits, vegetables, nuts and seeds. The diet was low in carbohydrates and relatively high in fat. It sounded interesting, so I ordered Robb Wolf's seminal book, **The Paleo Solution**, from Amazon, and we were on our way!

Little did I know that the Low Carb Flu season was just around the corner for me. I had read about the Low Carb Flu—it was essentially a withdrawal from carbohydrate addiction. Before I could reap the rewards of living a Paleo lifestyle, I would have to pay the price for my long-standing relationship with pasta, rice, bread and crackers. Especially crackers.

Symptoms of the Low Carb Flu included increased tiredness, worsening low blood sugar attacks, cravings for sugary or carbohydrate-laden foods, irritability, poor concentration, and headaches. Most people, I read, overcame these symptoms in a week or two. Extreme cases could last up to three weeks.

Bill and I commenced our excursion into feeling lousy together. We ate high protein, high fat, low carbohydrate meals and eliminated sugar from our diets altogether, while we continued to feed our four children the carbohydrates to which they were accustomed. At night, alone in our bedroom, we commiserated about how awful we felt. Together, we looked forward to sunnier, happier days of looking and feeling great together.

After about a week, Bill was no longer feeling ill, and he was starting to lose weight. I, on the other hand, hadn't lost a single pound, and I was feeling worse than ever. I wanted to throttle him, as he crooned about his loosening pants. My hypoglycemic attacks were becoming more frequent, and more severe. Some days, I could barely get out of bed, I was so fatigued. I consoled myself with the certainty that the malaise would soon be over.

Another week of misery passed. Then another. It had been a month since we started. I was just beginning to think that I must be the only person in the world for whom the Paleo Diet wouldn't work. Then the bacon cravings came. I didn't know it at the time, but my deliverance was about to make its appearance.

"This is crazy," I thought, as I put the sixth slice of thick-cut bacon into the frying pan. "Nobody can eat like this and live to tell about it." Yet all I could think about, night and day, was bacon. My body was screaming at me, "Feed me bacon!" and all I could do was obey. Day after day, I ate half a pound or more of bacon. And miracle of miracles—I started feeling better!

I felt like doing things again, only now, I found that I could go seven or eight hours without food. Before going Paleo, I was a wreck if I didn't eat within half an hour of getting up in the morning, and every two or three hours all day long. After the end of the Low Carb Flu episode, I noticed that for several days, four o'clock p.m. came and went without my falling apart from low blood sugar.

I had made an appointment with an endocrinologist several weeks earlier to discuss these distressing hypoglycemic attacks. By the day of the appointment, I felt as if I didn't even need to go, because I had stopped suffering from low blood sugar. I decided to keep the appointment, just to see what the doctor would say about my bacon-heavy diet.

"I'm not really having low blood sugar attacks anymore," I told the doctor, as she tested my sugar level. "I feel so much better. I've changed my diet a lot."

"What are you doing differently?" she asked.

Somewhat sheepishly, I told her, "I have drastically increased my dietary fat." I expected her to whirl around and prick me to death with the blood sugar tester. I certainly didn't expect the reaction that I got.

"Really?" Glowing smile, shining eyes. "Who told you that you should do that?"

"I, uh, sort of figured it out by myself." I mumbled.

"Well, you did exactly the right thing! Keep on eating good fats in abundance, and you just might cure yourself of hypoglycemia forever." She was looking at me like I was a genius. I was starting to feel like a genius, actually. I straightened my shoulders and mentally patted myself on the back for being a natural-born nutrition prodigy.

Except, of course, that I wasn't. I hadn't invented something new; I was just following a diet that had been discovered by someone else. I started to lose weight. At first, I wore a size 14 jeans. Then, I shrunk to a 12. Then a size 10, and an 8. I completely skipped size 6 and went straight to wearing a size 4, when the 8s got too big.

And I wasn't suffering. I didn't feel deprived. I ate as much as I wanted, whenever I was hungry—of certain foods. I ate chocolate **every single day**! I knew that I would have to be careful not to become a Paleo Diet zealot and risk driving all of my friends away. I wanted to tell the world that I had found, not just **a** new way of eating, but **the** way to eat for better all-round quality of life. One day, I realized that I never had to worry again about being fat. It was a quiet, but certain, moment of victory.

That's my story. And it's why I'm here to tell you about living Paleo, for good.

Conclusion

Not everybody will undertake Paleo living and stick with it. But everybody would be better off, if they did. I firmly believe that the Paleo Diet and its accompanying lifestyle shifts have the power to make every person on the planet healthier. If all folks went Paleo, blood pressure would go down, cancer would decrease, heart attacks would be fewer, diabetes would be a bye-gone problem...

Western society is so hooked on simple carbohydrates, though, that our world would be in a lot of collective pain, if everyone went Paleo at once. I can almost hear the collective groans...governments would grind to a screeching halt, bombs would be dropped, and that would be just the beginning. The possessor of a jelly donut could sell it for a million dollars.

Clearly, a successful path to Paleo will not be pain-free. That will be the sticking point for some people reading this book. We are a comfort-loving people, and part of our cultural legacy is that we practically feel entitled to live a pain-free life.

The myth of a pain-free life, however, is just that—a myth. We may try to avoid pain, but it inevitably finds us, anyway.

Thus, the pertinent question is not, "Will I experience pain?" but rather, "**When** will I experience pain, and **what kind** of pain will it be?" The choice is ours to make; it isn't easy, but it is simple. We can avoid the pain of changing our diets now, and pay a huge price of pain later, when stress and disease catch up with us. Or we can embrace a relatively minor amount of pain now, make the transition to the Paleo Diet now, and reap a lifetime of the benefits of comfort stemming from radiant health.

It really boils down to changing short-term thinking (and gratification) into long-term thinking. If you buy better quality food, your grocery bill will go up, and you will probably have to cut back somewhere else in your budget to accommodate the increase. But 15 years from now, you will be able to spend your money on college for your children, vacations, a satisfying retirement—you fill in the blanks—instead of high-priced medical procedures, drugs with bad side effects and wheelchairs.

So, it's not a matter of, "Will I pay?" but rather a matter of, "Will I pay now or later?"

One parting thought to contemplate: Is it possible that, just maybe, the fear of pain is worse than pain itself? Hmm...